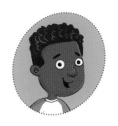

In Our Neighborhood

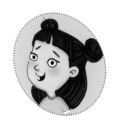

Meet a Nurse!

by Cyndy Unwin

Illustrations by Lisa Hunt

Children's Press®
An imprint of Scholastic Inc.

SCHOLASTIC

Special thanks to our content consultants:

Emelie Moles, RN
Oak Grove Elementary School
Roanoke, VA

Rachel McLaughlin, RN

Library of Congress Cataloging-in-Publication Data
Names: Unwin, Cyndy, author. | Hunt, Lisa, 1973– illustrator.
Title: Meet a nurse!/by Cyndy Unwin; [illustrations by Lisa Hunt.]
Other titles: Meet a nurse!
Description: New York: Children's Press, an imprint of Scholastic Inc., 2021. | Series: In our neighborhood |
    Includes index. | Audience: Ages 5–7. | Audience: Grades K–1. | Summary: "This book introduces readers
    to the role of nurses in their community"— Provided by publisher.
Identifiers: LCCN 2020033786 | ISBN 9780531136850 (library binding) | ISBN 9780531136911 (paperback)
Subjects: LCSH: Nurses—Juvenile literature. | Nursing—Juvenile literature.
Classification: LCC RT61.5 .U59 2021 | DDC 610.73—dc23
LC record available at https://lccn.loc.gov/2020033786

Produced by Spooky Cheetah Press
Prototype design by Maria Bergós/Book & Look
Page design by Kathleen Petelinsek/The Design Lab

Printed in North Mankato, MN, USA 113

SCHOLASTIC, CHILDREN'S PRESS, IN OUR NEIGHBORHOOD™, and associated
logos are trademarks and/or registered trademarks of Scholastic Inc.

1 2 3 4 5 6 7 8 9 10 R 30 29 28 27 26 25 24 23 22 21

Scholastic Inc., 557 Broadway, New York, NY 10012.

Photos ©: 7: Ariel Skelley/Getty Images; 11: Mladen Sladojevic/Getty Images;
13: SDI Productions/Getty Images; 14: Richard Green/Alamy Images;
16 left: FatCamera/Getty Images; 16 right: Hispanolistic/Getty Images;
17 right: South_agency/Getty Images; 19: SDI Productions/Getty Images;
22: sturti/Getty Images; 25: FatCamera/Getty Images; 31 top right: Science
Source; 31 bottom left: Mihailvb/Dreamstime.

All other photos © Shutterstock.

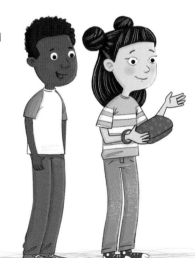

Table of Contents

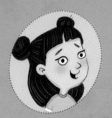

OUR NEIGHBORHOOD

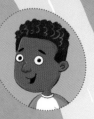

Hi! I'm Emma. This is my best friend, Theo. Welcome to our neighborhood!

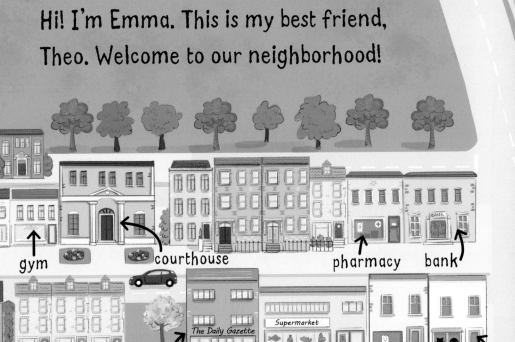

gym

courthouse

pharmacy

bank

The Daily Gazette

local newspaper

Supermarket

supermarket

dentist

veterinarian

salon

movie theater

POLICE STATION

police station

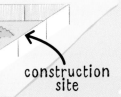

construction site

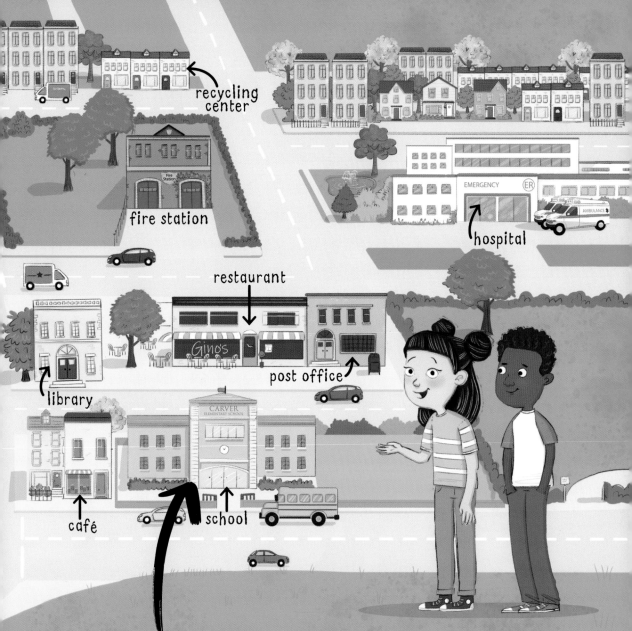

Our school is right over there. We have the greatest school nurse, Mr. Henry. Theo and I have been learning about how much he helps us every day!

MEET NURSE HENRY

Last Friday, we were playing freeze tag in gym class. All of a sudden, I couldn't breathe. Ms. Adams called Nurse Henry on her walkie-talkie. He helped me calm down and catch my breath.

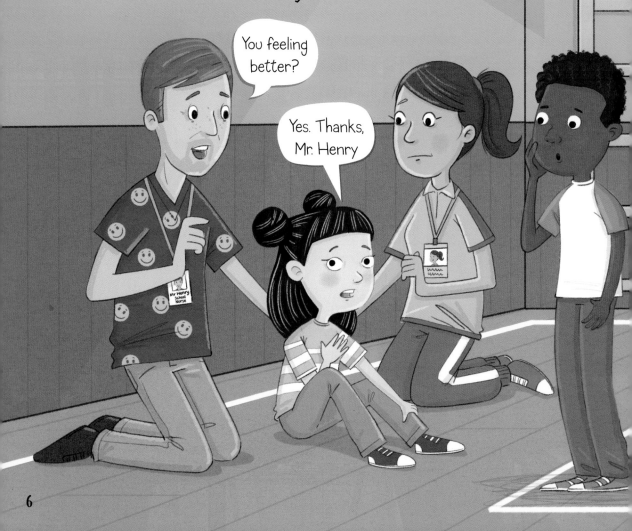

Mr. Henry said I should see my doctor, so my mom picked me up early from school.

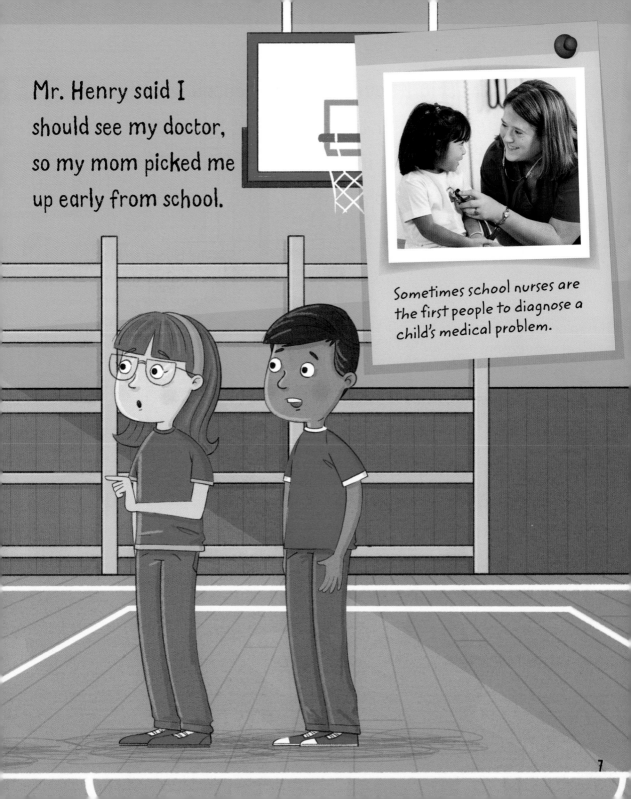

Sometimes school nurses are the first people to diagnose a child's medical problem.

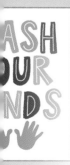

My doctor said I have exercise-induced asthma and gave me an inhaler to use before gym. She told me to keep the inhaler in the nurse's office. My mom came with me to school on Monday morning to drop it off.

I'll make sure Emma is using her inhaler correctly.

NORMAL AIRWAY

ASTHMATIC AIRWAY

If you have asthma, the tubes bringing air into and out of your lungs can become narrow. That can make breathing difficult.

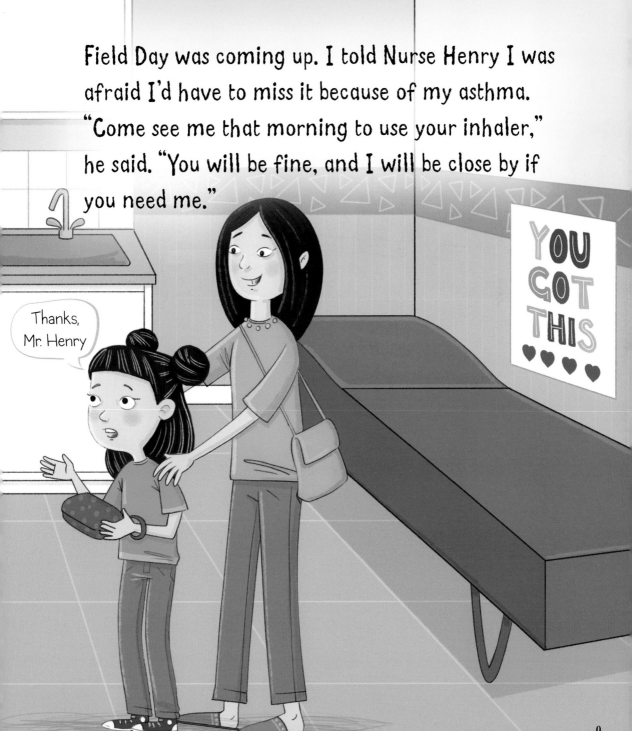

Field Day was coming up. I told Nurse Henry I was afraid I'd have to miss it because of my asthma. "Come see me that morning to use your inhaler," he said. "You will be fine, and I will be close by if you need me."

Thanks, Mr. Henry

On Wednesday, we had gym class after lunch. I asked Theo to come with me to the nurse's office to get my asthma treatment. We were just leaving the cafeteria when our friend Sophie hurried over to us. She looked worried.

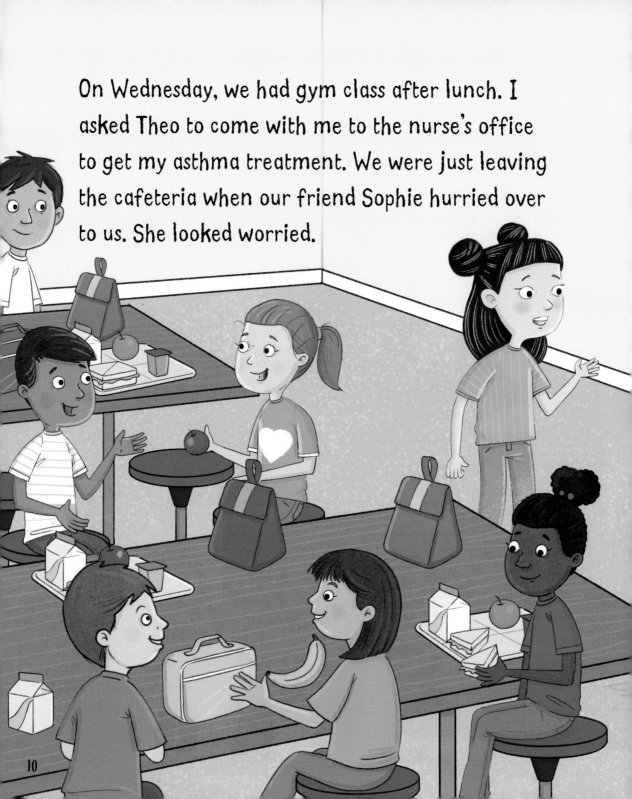

Sophie told us she had eaten something that made her mouth tingle. She was afraid she was having an allergic reaction. Sophie and one of the teachers on cafeteria duty came with us to see Mr. Henry. Nurse Henry gave Sophie her medicine, and she started to feel better right away.

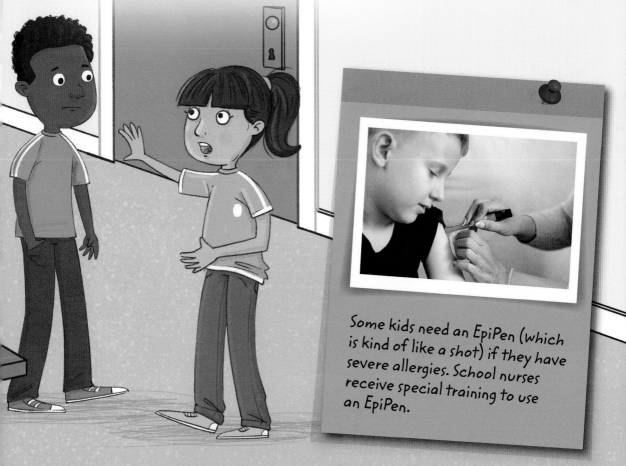

Some kids need an EpiPen (which is kind of like a shot) if they have severe allergies. School nurses receive special training to use an EpiPen.

We were getting ready for Field Day, so gym class was outside that day. Theo and I practiced tug-of-war. I was really happy that my inhaler worked. I felt great! But Theo got some splinters in his finger from the thick rope.

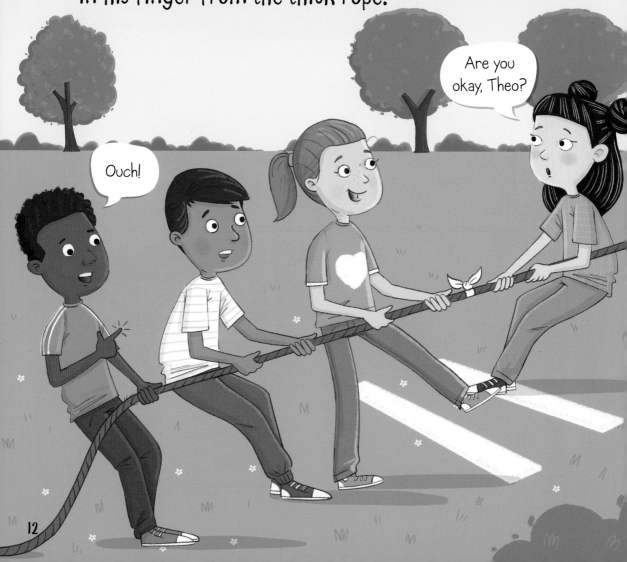

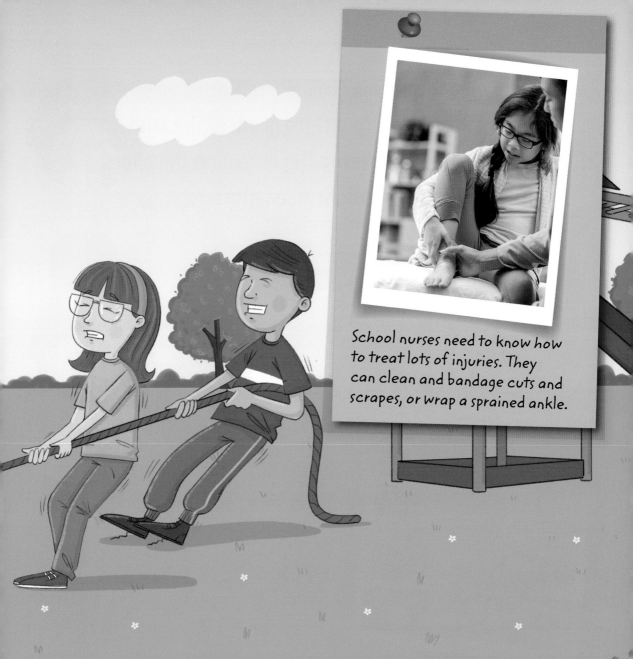

School nurses need to know how to treat lots of injuries. They can clean and bandage cuts and scrapes, or wrap a sprained ankle.

We went back to the nurse's office AGAIN so Nurse Henry could take out the splinters with his tweezers.

When we got to his office, Nurse Henry was giving a vision test to a third grader. The student was having trouble seeing the letters on the chart. Mr. Henry said she might need glasses.

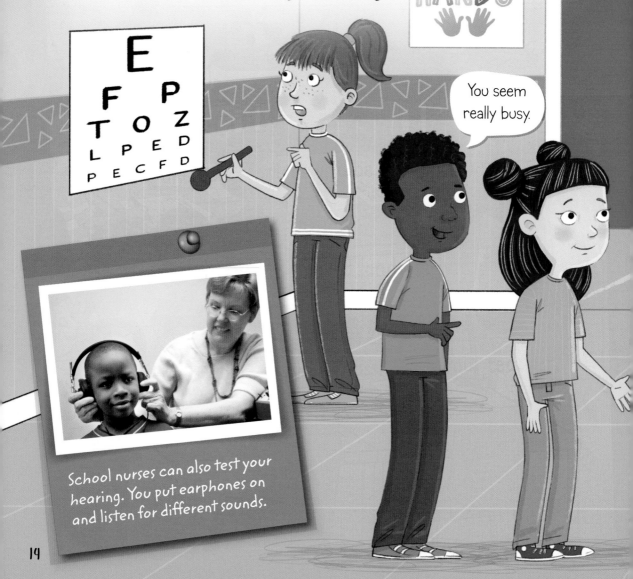

You seem really busy.

School nurses can also test your hearing. You put earphones on and listen for different sounds.

Then our friend Eli came in. He had just lost his first tooth. Mr. Henry helped Eli rinse out his mouth. He gave Eli a little treasure chest to take his tooth home in.

I am. But I always have time for you!

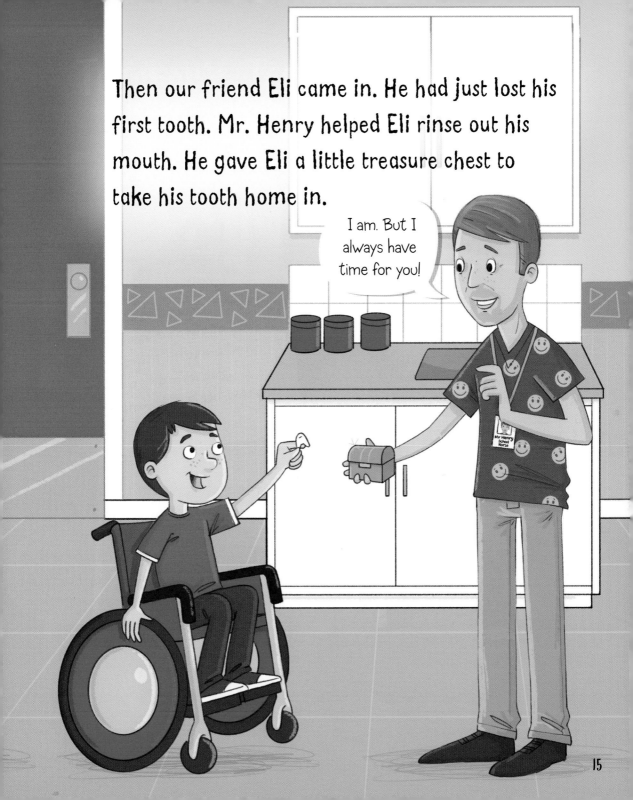

Mr. Henry told us being a school nurse keeps him very busy. Theo asked him what other types of jobs nurses have. "Nurses work in all sorts of places," Mr. Henry said.

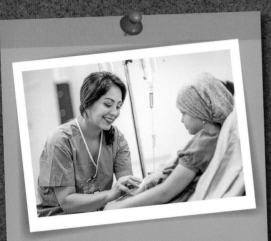

Hospital nurses take care of patients who are sick or have had an operation.

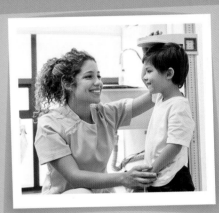

Pediatric nurses might take a child's temperature or check their height and weight before they see their doctor for a checkup.

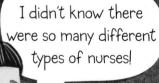

I didn't know there were so many different types of nurses!

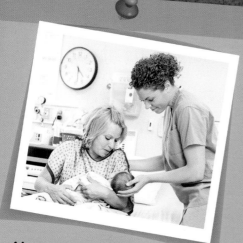

Neonatal nurses work in the newborn nursery in a hospital. They help babies and their parents.

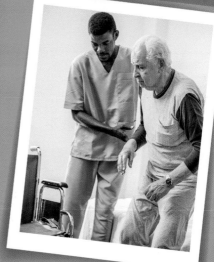

Geriatric nurses take care of elderly people.

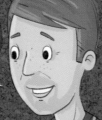

Each nursing job takes special training.

17

Finally, Field Day was just one day away! Nurse Henry visited our classroom to talk to us about being safe. He told us to wear sunscreen and drink lots of water. He also reminded me to come to his office to use my inhaler before the events start.

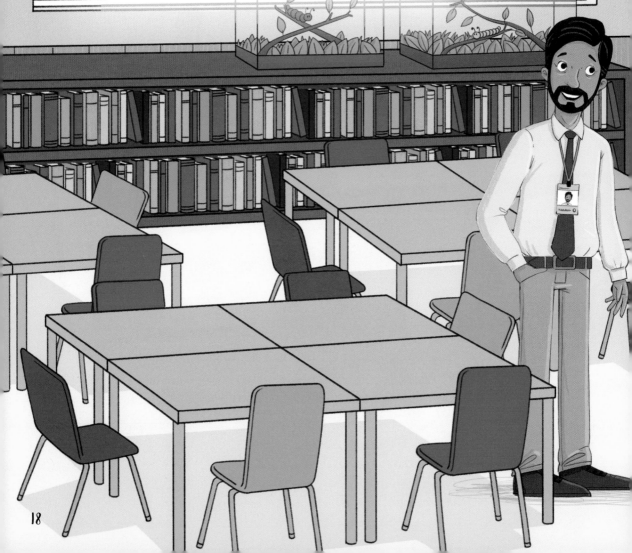

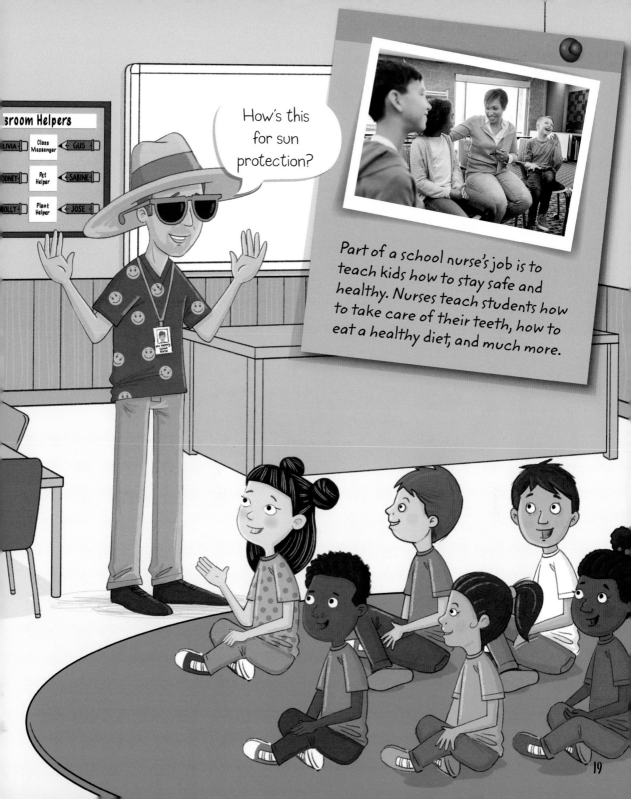

How's this for sun protection?

Part of a school nurse's job is to teach kids how to stay safe and healthy. Nurses teach students how to take care of their teeth, how to eat a healthy diet, and much more.

19

FIELD DAY!

Field Day was a LOT of fun . . . until I got to the obstacle course. I was almost to the finish line when I started having trouble breathing.

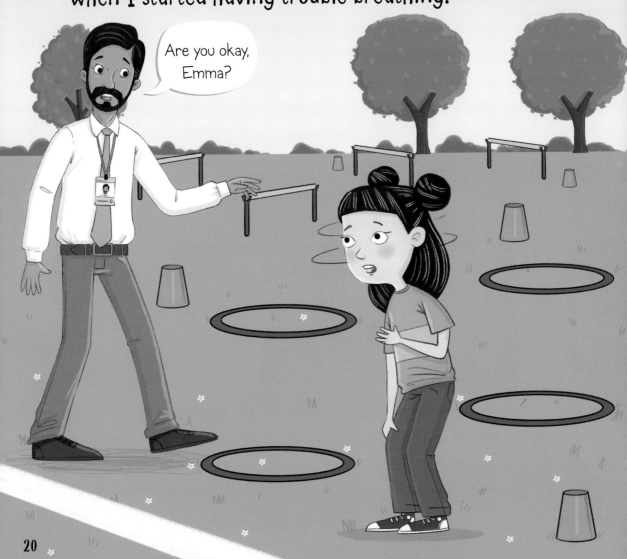

Are you okay, Emma?

I stopped and tried to take a deep breath, but I felt worse and worse. I was starting to feel afraid.

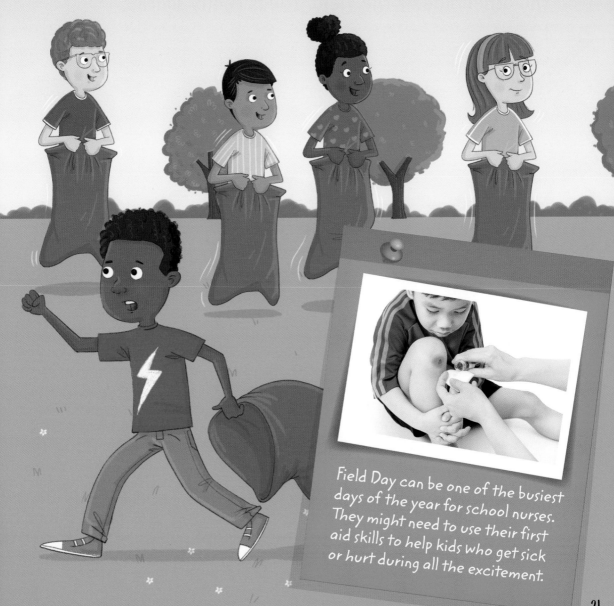

Field Day can be one of the busiest days of the year for school nurses. They might need to use their first aid skills to help kids who get sick or hurt during all the excitement.

Theo and my teacher helped me walk to the first aid station. My teacher waved my mom over from the other side of the field. I was really scared.

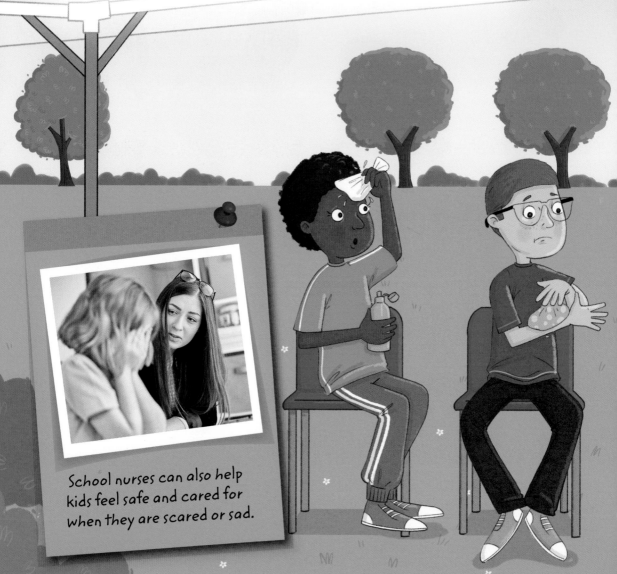

School nurses can also help kids feel safe and cared for when they are scared or sad.

Nurse Henry came over right away with my inhaler. He made sure I used it correctly and then listened to my lungs. He sat with me until I felt calmer.

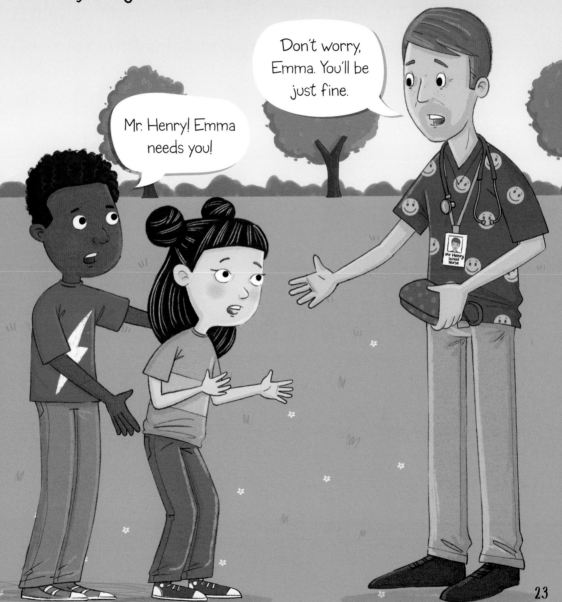

Mr. Henry! Emma needs you!

Don't worry, Emma. You'll be just fine.

23

BREATHING EASY

I started to feel better after a few minutes, but I could tell my mom was still a little worried. I told her how much Nurse Henry had helped me.

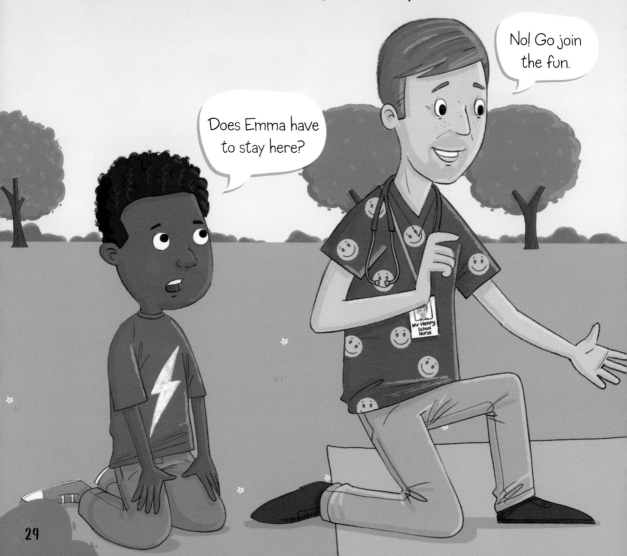

"Mr. Henry, you do so much for this school," my mom said. "Thank you for everything you've done for Emma, too!"

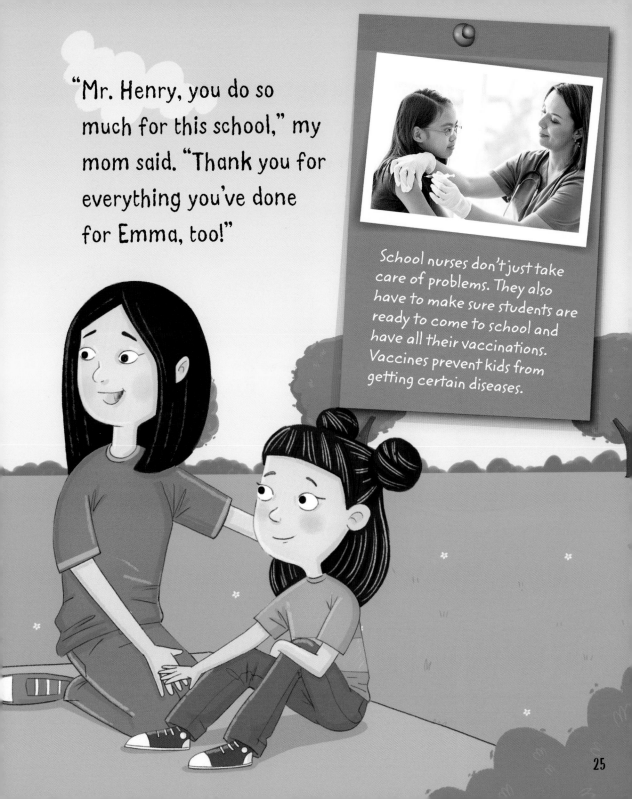

School nurses don't just take care of problems. They also have to make sure students are ready to come to school and have all their vaccinations. Vaccines prevent kids from getting certain diseases.

Field Day was over, and the teachers were handing out ice pops. Theo chose cherry, and I picked my favorite—orange. Then we went to sit with the rest of our class.

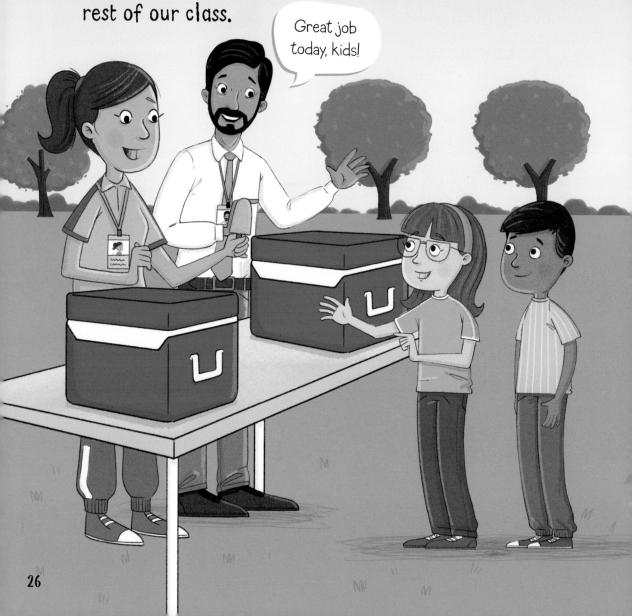

Great job today, kids!

We'd all done really well in the events. But, most important, we had a lot of fun. Even me . . . now that I was feeling better!

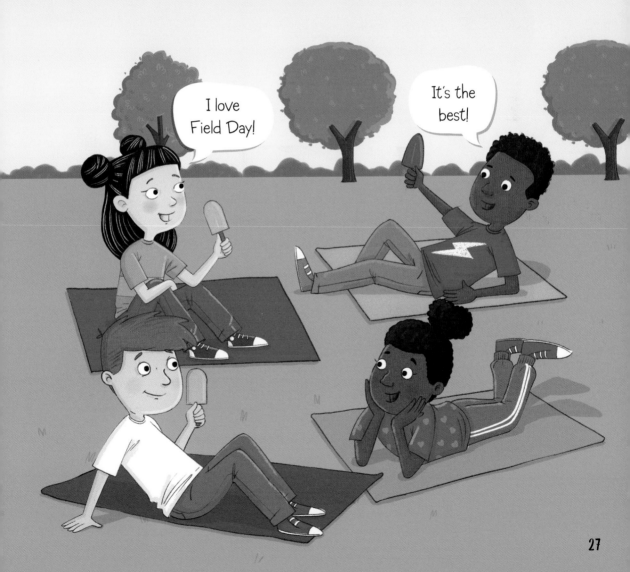

Ask a School Nurse

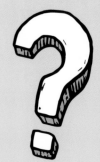

Theo asked Nurse Henry some questions at the end of the day.

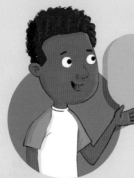

If I wanted to be a nurse, what kind of schooling would I need?

There are many kinds of nurses. Most school nurses are registered nurses, or RNs. To become an RN, you need at least two years of college, and you have to pass a test.

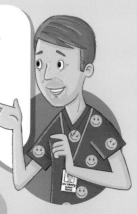

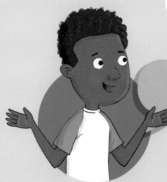

What's your favorite part of your job?

I love going into classrooms and teaching kids about staying healthy.

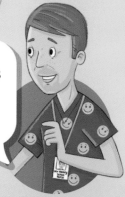

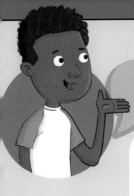

How do you help kids in our school?

School nurses make sure kids are taking their medicines correctly. We can check your vision and hearing. We do first aid if you are hurt or sick. And we care for kids who have medical problems like diabetes, asthma, or allergies.

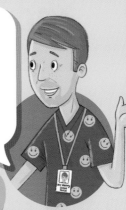

What do you do besides take care of sick kids?

We check your hair and scalp and help if you have an itchy problem with head lice. We can also check your spine to make sure it's curving the right way as you grow.

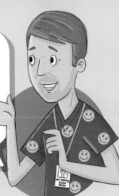

Do we have to be sick or hurt to come see you?

No! School nurses love it when students stop by the office to say hi. We're also really good listeners if something's bothering you. Just make sure you have your teacher's permission to visit!

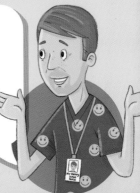

Nurse Henry's Health and Safety Tips

- Less screen time, more feet time! You need 60 minutes of physical activity every day.

- Eat five to nine servings of fruits and vegetables every day. Don't eat too much sugar!

- Wear sunscreen when you swim or play outdoors.

- Always have an adult with you when you swim.

- Remember to drink lots of water when you're playing—especially if it's hot outside. Don't wait until you're thirsty!

- Stranger danger! If someone you don't know approaches you, follow the "No, Go, Yell, Tell" rule: Say no, run away, yell as loud as you can, and tell a trusted adult what happened.

A School Nurse's Tools

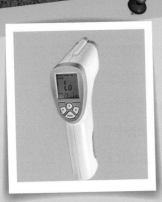

Thermometer: Nurses use this tool to measure a patient's temperature.

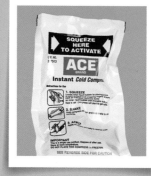

Ice packs: Nurses use ice packs to keep pain and swelling down.

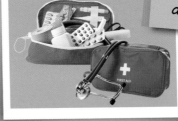

First aid supplies: These are the items nurses use to treat minor cuts, bruises, scrapes, and burns.

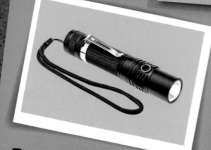

Flashlight: Nurses can use a flashlight to look at your throat if it's sore.

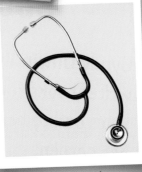

Stethoscope: Nurses use this instrument to listen to the heart and lungs.

Index

About the Author

Cyndy Unwin lives in the mountains of Virginia. She writes books for kids and is also a reading teacher. She loves eating berry-flavored ice pops after a hot day in her garden!